MW01506338

Growing Green Families

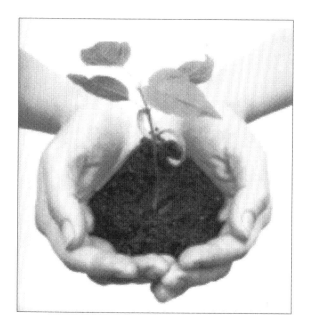

Donna Walls

RN, BSN, IBCLC, ICCE, ANLC

Master Herbalist,

Certified Aromatherapist

Praeclarus Press, LLC

www.PraeclarusPress.com

Praeclarus Press, LLC
2504 Sweetgum Lane
Amarillo, Texas 79124 USA
806-367-9950
www.PraeclarusPress.com

DISCLAIMER
The information contained in this publication is advisory only and is not intended to replace sound clinical judgment or individualized patient care. The author disclaims all warranties, whether expressed or implied, including any warranty as the quality, accuracy, safety, or suitability of this information for any particular purpose.

ISBN: 978-1-9398075-7-1

Cover Design and Production: Ken Tackett
Copy Editing: Chris Tackett
Acquisition & Development: Kathleen Kendall-Tackett
Layout & Design: Cornelia Georgiana Murariu

About the Author

My love affair with Mother Nature began while growing up in the 60s, a time when "getting back to nature" was the norm. Respecting the natural world, and living in a harmonious way with the rhythms and cycles of life, made a lot of sense to me. This way of thinking and living was always comfortable for me.

I finished nursing school in the early 70s, indoctrinated into Western medicine, and lived there for several years, during which time my babies were born, of course coming into the world naturally.

Having children changes you. It makes you more protective, and more vigilant. I always called it the Mother Wolf way guarding your babies. I questioned the standard ways of healing and chose a more natural healing system for them, including having no chips and pop in the house—sometimes not a popular decision.

The children grew healthy and strong, and soon they were out on their own, a difficult, but normal, loving separation. The time that was once filled with laundry and carpooling was mine/ours for the first time.

I felt those first stirrings of that dormant passion for all things natural again, and felt the need to live everyday in the forgotten rhythms of life. I became a Master Herbalist, opening a practice quietly to spread the gospel of herbal and natural healing. It was congruent with my work as a nurse, in which I had chosen to support natural birth choices by opening an "alternative" birth center, and continued to support breastfeeding as a lactation consultant.

My life became greener, expanding into teaching (and preaching) about the glories of natural cleaning, natural and herbal healing, and healthy food choices. My husband, family, and friends listened politely. Some even heard.

So here I am, mid-life now, with a burning need to have more people listen, have more people hear, and have more people take action. Hopefully, this book will help others on this path for a cleaner, healthier planet.

Dedication

To my husband, Don, for his unfailing support of my dreams,

To my daughter, Sara, for believing in and living the vision,

To my son, Eric, who loves and respects nature,

To my stepson, Derek, who chooses to live in the beauty of the mountains,

To Cindy Puskar, Susan Bash, Anne Brower, and all my friends for listening,

and

For a greener, healthier world for my grandchildren,

Macey, Madeline, Eli, Bella, Nolan, and Laney.

Contents

Introduction

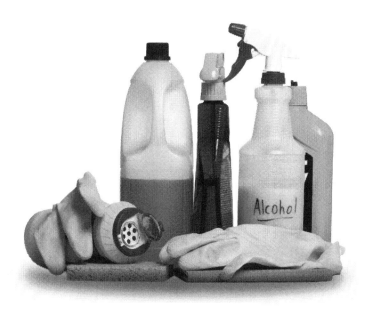

It's in the news, on the radio, and in newspapers and magazines; there's a concern about the effects of so many chemicals and pollutants on our health. We are constantly being bombarded with toxic chemicals in our food, the air, and our water supply.

> What can you do?

> March with "Save our Earth" signs?

> Donate to environmental defense groups?

> Send out informational emails and use social media to let everyone know?

Yes, all of these actions are good. But the best place to start is at home with your family. We can make our little corners of the world a little better, a little safer, a little kinder.

Becoming aware of potentially harmful chemicals is the first step.

Which chemicals, additives, or substances do we need to remove (or recycle) from our homes?

How can we remove them safely?

What are the best alternatives to "get the job done?"

Even more important; how can we become aware, take action, and not let ourselves become so vigilant, so aware, so motivated, and so afraid, that we forget to enjoy the beauty of the Earth around us, the sounds of our children and grandchildren laughing, the calm of music softly playing, and living our best life?

What do we need to do to make our homes and families safer? First, educate yourself and your family about the chemicals that may be of concern. Second, take action to choose and use healthier alternatives.

It All Starts with Pregnancy

How can we keep pregnancy cleaner, safer, and healthier?

In 2013, the American College of Obstetricians and Gynecologists and the American Society for Reproductive Medicine released a joint statement that said "toxic chemicals in our environment harm our ability to reproduce, negatively affect pregnancies, and are associated with numerous long-term health problems."

Talk with your doctor or midwife about how to protect yourself and your baby from harmful environmental substances. Here are a few suggestions:

Xenoestrogens. Xenoestrogrens are often referred to as environmental estrogens. They are man-made chemicals that are very similar to the female hormone estrogen. They react very differently in the body from natural hormones and cause unusual responses. These chemical are associated with increasing rates of reproductive cancers, fetal abnormalities, chromosomal damage, and numerous other health hazards—many in the developing fetus.

How can women who are planning to become pregnant, or who are pregnant, avoid exposures to these environmental estrogens?

> Minimize or avoid the use of plastics for preparing, serving, or storing foods.

> Use only non-toxic, chemical-free household cleaners. (EWG.org/cleaningguides)

> Purchase and prepare organic, hormone-free foods as much as possible. Also, avoid GMO foods, artificial sweeteners, and artificial preservatives and dyes.

> Use basic, natural personal care products. (EWG.org/skindeep)

> Avoid the use of lawn and garden care herbicides and pesticides.

> Consider installing a water filter to avoid ingestion of lead and other toxic chemicals.

> Avoid fish species known to be high in mercury: king mackerel, marlin, orange roughy, shark, swordfish, tilefish, ahi tuna, and bigeye tuna. For more information go to https://www.nrdc.org/stories/smart-seafood-buying-guide.

> Educate yourself on safe products for infant supplies and infant care.

Harmful Household Chemicals

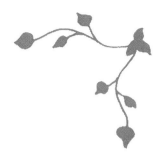

There is good reason to be concerned about the harmful effects of commercially produced cleaning products. In our zeal to keep the germs at bay, we have created a more hazardous environment with the chemicals than the threat from the bad bugs.

Both the Children's Health Environmental Coalition and the Healthcare Environmental Resource Center, recommend a simple, common sense approach: minimize exposure to chemical cleaners and use safer, natural alternatives whenever possible!

To help you select household cleaning products that are safer, look for the Green Seal, or the EcoLogo. Both organizations provide certifications for environmentally friendly cleaners. For information to help you choose products, you can go to http://www.ewg.org/guides/cleaners.

The *Dirty Dozen* List of Chemicals Known to Contribute to Cancer Development

In 2015, the Environmental Working Group published the *Dirty Dozen* of chemicals known to contribute to cancer development:

1. **BPA** found in canned food linings, polycarbonate (#7) plastics, and on paper receipts.

2. **Atrazine:** a widely used herbicide

3. **Organophosphate Pesticides.** Another good reason to choose organic foods.

4. **Dibutyl Phthalate (DBP):** used in plastics.

5. **Lead,** often found in older chipping paints, and in some water sources.

6. **Mercury,** found in fish. See the EWG seafood calculator.

7. **PFCs** (polyflurochemicals) found in stain replants and non-stick cookware.

8. **Phthalates,** found in plastics, soft vinyl toys, and extended use fragrances.

9. **Diethlyhexyl Phthalate (DEHP),** often found in synthetic fragrances, and plastic foodware.

10. **PDBEs** are flame retardants used before 2005 in foam, clothing, and furniture.

11. **Triclosan,** an antibacterial used in soaps and sanitizers.

12. **Nonylphenol,** used in detergents and personal care products.

Other Chemicals on the *Use with Great Caution* List

1. **Chlorine bleach** causes respiratory damage and eye irritation, and is a known carcinogen.

2. **Petroleum distillates** damage the lungs, kidneys, eyes, and the central nervous system.

3. **Perchloroethylene (PERC)** is toxic to the central nervous system.

4. **Ammonia** irritates the eyes and lungs, and is linked to headaches.

5. **Phenol and Creosols** in disinfectants cause kidney and liver damage.

6. **Nitrobenzenes** in floor and furniture polishes are linked to cancer and birth defects.

7. **Formaldehyde** is used as a preservative in many household cleaners, and is added to bedding for a wrinkle-free finish, is linked to cancer and is an irritant to eyes, throat, skin, and lungs.

8. **Naphthalene** in mothballs is damaging to kidneys, liver, skin, and the central nervous system.

9. **Hydrochloric or Sodium Acid Sulfate** in toilet bowl cleaners is caustic to skin, eyes, and lungs.

Cleaning with a Conscience

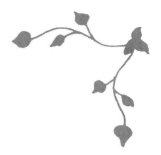

Keep your home clean with some kitchen cupboard basics:

> **Vinegar** sanitizes and removes stains.

> **Lemon juice** works safely to disinfect.

> **Baking soda** is a great all-purpose cleaner.

> **Borax** is an all-natural cleanser.

> **Cornstarch** is an easy, natural de-greaser.

> **Olive oil** is great for dusting and furniture polishing.

> **Grapefruit seed extract** is a natural germ killer.

> **Pure essential oils** are natural germ killers and natural fragrances.

> **Herbal infusions** are natural fragrances.

With these basic ingredients, you can clean almost any surface in your home!

Baking Soda Cleaning

🍃 To unclog kitchen drains, pour ½ cup baking soda into drain, follow with ½ cup white vinegar. After foaming stops, follow with 1 quart boiling water

🍃 For sweat stains, add water to baking soda to form a paste, rub into stain, and allow to sit for 10 to 15 minutes. Launder as usual.

- 🌿 For safely cleaning ovens, spray oven surfaces with water and sprinkle with baking soda. Allow to sit overnight. Re-spray with water and wipe clean.

- 🌿 Add 2 to 3 tablespoons baking soda, and a squirt of any natural dishwashing soap, to dish water to soak food-dried dishes, pots, and pans.

- 🌿 To freshen sponges, work baking soda well into a wet sponge. For extra cleaning, place sponge in the top rack of the dishwasher or place in microwave for 30 to 40 seconds.

- 🌿 For non-abrasive microwave cleaning, place a small amount of baking soda on a damp cloth or sponge. Clean as usual, and rinse well.

- 🌿 For easy carpet deodorizing, sprinkle baking soda on the carpet, allow to sit overnight, and vacuum the next day.

- 🌿 Deodorize your refrigerator by leaving an opened box of baking soda in the refrigerator.

Vinegar Cleaning

- 🌿 Add 1/2 cup white vinegar to the final rinse for a natural fabric softener.

- 🌿 To reduce that "vinegar" smell, simmer aromatic herbs for 15 to 20 minutes in the vinegar, strain out the plants, and then use as fabric softener.

- 🌿 Remove perspiration odors and stains by spraying the area with full strength white vinegar, allow to set about 5 minutes, and add to usual laundry.

- To clean coffee pots, fill with warm water, and add ½ cup vinegar and 1 tsp baking soda. Allow to "fizz" and rinse clean.

- For sparkling windows, add ¼ cup vinegar to 2 cups water, and wipe with soft cloth or unbleached paper towels.

- For general cleaning, mix equal parts of distilled water and white vinegar. Store in a spritzer bottle for easy use.

Lemon Juice Cleaning

- Dilute lemon juice with half juice and half water to remove waxes and pesticide residue on produce.

- To clean cutting boards, cut a lemon in half and scrub directly with the raw lemon or use undiluted lemon juice.

Coarse Salt for Abrasive Cleaning

- When rust or built-up food accumulates, scrub with coarse salt.

Making Herbal Infusions for Cleaning Solutions

- Heat 1 cup water to simmering (not boiling). Add 1 to 2 tablespoon dried organic herbs, and steep for 10 to 15 minutes. Strain out plant material and allow to cool. Store in dark glass jars for best storage. If you are preparing infusions for later use, distilled water will increase the length of storage times.

Herbs especially helpful in making cleaning infusions:

> Lavender   > Sage   > Dried lemon
> Rosemary   > Oregano   or orange
             > Thyme   rinds

Add these infusions to water or vinegar solutions for germ killing and a clean, fresh smell.

Using Essential Oils for Cleaning

These plant extracts are very concentrated, and recipes will call for only drops. "If a little bit is good, a lot is better" *does not* apply here! Because of their high concentration, they need to be diluted before coming into contact with the skin.

Essential oils blend well with base oils, like olive or wheat germ oil, for furniture polishing. But if diluting essential oils in water for liquid cleaners and spritzers, add a small amount of witch hazel to help mix the oils in the water.

Some of the essential oils used commonly in cleaning products are:

> Lemon
> Orange
> Mints
> Lavender
> Tea tree

They are all great germ-killers, and also leave a fresher, less *toxic* smell in the air.

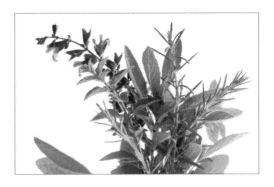

The Recipes for a Cleaner Home, Naturally

Lemon & Mint Window Cleaner

Juice from 1 lemon (1/4 cup lemon juice)
2 cups water
10 drops peppermint essential oil

🌿 Mix well and place in spray bottle, clean as usual

Toilet Bowl Spray Cleaner

2 tablespoons each of vinegar and baking soda mixed well in 2 cups water
Add 1 teaspoon grapefruit seed extract and 10 drops orange essential oil and mix well.

🌿 After foaming stops, place in spray bottle. Spray in toilet bowl and clean with non-disposable toilet brush.

Moth Repellant

1 cup rosemary leaves
1 cup sage leaves
1 cup cedar shavings
5 bruised bay leaves

- 🍃 Mix well and place in cloth bags. Muslin works well.
- 🍃 Hang or place in needed areas.

Bug and Mouse Repellants

Ants: Sprinkle cinnamon, coffee grounds, or cornmeal in areas where ants appear.

Lemon juice mixed with water in a spray.

Vinegar spray

1 teaspoon boric acid
6 tablespoons sugar
2 cups water

- 🍃 Dissolve boric acid and sugar in water thoroughly. Soak cotton balls in the solution and place in paper bag with small holes punched in the sides.

- 🍃 Place in needed areas and change cotton balls once a week. Dispose of bags when filled with deceased varmints.

Fruit Flies: Pour a glass of sweet wine, add a drop of soap, and leave near the flies.

Spiders: Place hedge apples around the outside of the house.

Mice: Place peppermint essential oil in infested areas.

Cleaners

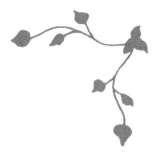

Kitchen Surface Cleanser

4 oz distilled water
4 oz white vinegar
1 tablespoon baking soda
15 to 20 drops of lavender or lemon essential oil

Dishwasher Spot Remover

Add white vinegar in the rinse compartment of your dishwasher.

To Clean Porcelain Surfaces

Wet a soft cloth and sprinkle with cream of tartar until the powder is *paste-like*. Clean and rinse as usual.

Sneaker Tamer

¼ cup corn starch
¼ cup baking soda
10 drops citrus essential oil

Sprinkle in shoes and allow to sit overnight whenever needed.

Pesky Pet Stain and Odor Destroyer

8 oz white vinegar
8 oz citrus rind infused distilled water
1 tablespoon each tea-tree and lemon pure essential oils

🌿 Mix well and place in a spray bottle. Spray directly on stain and work in well. Rinse and allow to dry. Repeat if necessary.

Freshening Closets or Drawers

🌿 In a small cloth or muslin bag, place equal parts of lavender, mint, lemon balm, and rose petals. Hang in closets or place in drawers to freshen clothing, blankets, and linens.

Air Freshening: Indoors

🌿 To avoid synthetic room deodorizers or plug-in scents, keep a bowl of pine needles, mint leaves, aromatic herbs, or flower buds wherever needed.

🌿 For bathroom freshening, place a few drops of sage, lavender, or lemon essential oil on the inside of the toilet paper roll.

Laundry Freshener

In a small muslin bag, place 1 teaspoon each of lavender buds, rosemary leaves, and sage leaves.

🌿 Toss into dryer cycle for fresh clothes.

Laundry Detergent

8 cups baking soda
6 cups borax
4 cups grated castile or glycerin soap
2 tablespoons lavender or citrus essential oil

🌿 Combine and mix well. Use ¼ to 1/3 cups per load.

🌿 For *bleaching*, use hydrogen peroxide or lemon juice.

Spot Remover for All Fabrics

🌿 Blend together 4 tablespoons liquid glycerin and 2 tablespoons borax to form a paste.

🌿 Work well into stain and wash as usual.

Thyme Furniture Wax

2 oz beeswax
12 oz thyme herbal infusion
1 oz olive or other vegetable oil
5 drops thyme essential oil

🌿 Heat 1 ½ cups distilled water to simmering. Place 1 to 2 tablespoons dried thyme leaves in water and steep for 15 minutes. Remove herbs.

🌿 Melt beeswax in hot thyme infusion. Add olive or other oil, and essential oil. Cool and store in dark glass bottle and clean furniture as usual.

Furniture Polish

1 cup olive or other natural vegetable oil
1 teaspoon lemon juice
5 drops lemon essential oil

🍃 Mix well and clean wooden furniture as usual.

Mold and Mildew Remover

2 cups distilled water
1 oz grapefruit seed extract
1 tablespoon tea-tree essential oil

🍃 Mix well and place in spray bottle. Spritz area and allow to sit on surface for 5 to 10 minutes before cleaning. Rinse and dry area.

Replacing shower curtains with natural fabrics, like cotton or hemp rather than the usual PVC plastic liner, reduces mold growth, makes shower curtains machine washable, and reduces off-gassing of harmful vapors.

Also, keep bathroom windows open whenever weather permits, for better ventilation and natural sunlight, to reduce the growth of mold and mildew.

Recycling

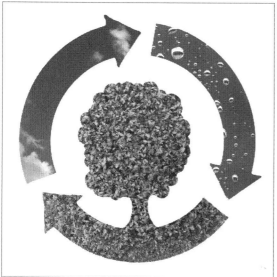

Don't forget about recycling in your home. Find out about your local recycling options and make it a part of your daily routine. When purchasing supplies for your family, choose recycled products whenever possible.

Avoid the trap of all those convenient disposables for cleaning. Sounds so tempting to just wipe and throw away. But where are all those conveniences going? How many landfills or toxic burns are used to "get rid of" the cleverly marketed supplies? Reusing old towels, diapers, t-shirts, or any cloth rags can make a huge impact on the environment.

Remember to wash the kitchen dish cloths frequently in hot, soapy water, and/or soak in vinegar to prevent the growth of mold and germs.

Avoid using plastic grocery bags. Better to reuse paper bags for as long as they can be used. Or even better, use canvas bags for shopping.

If every household replaced their paper towels with recycled paper towels, we could save 1.2 million trees and 3.7 million cubic feet of landfill space, and prevent 894 pounds of pollution. Think about how much more we could save by using and reusing cloth towels!

Earth911.org offers information on local recycling options.

Other Ways to Recycle and Help Others at the Same Time

> **Eyeglasses:** onesight.org

> **Cell phones:** cellphonesforsoldiers.com

> **Musical instruments:** therootsofmusic.com

> **Paint, tools, and building supplies:** habitat.org

> **Sports equipment:** sportsgift.org

> **Furniture and household goods:** goodwill.org or salvationarmyusa.org

Plastics. They are Everywhere! What are the Concerns?

Research from several consumer protection agencies have shown many of the "plasticizers," such as dioxin and bisphenol A (BPA), to be hormone disrupters, and known carcinogens. Plastic bottles, food wraps, storage containers, and storage bags are everywhere. It's hard to find food storage, or food preparation supplies not made of plastic.

How can we use plastics safely?

Do not use plastics when heating foods in the microwave. Avoid serving or storing hot foods in plastic containers. Research shows that heating releases these harmful chemicals that leach into the food.

- When heating foods, use ceramic or glass dishes covered with a plate or unbleached paper towel.

- Do not store bottled water or other beverages in garages or other areas that are not temperature controlled.

- Use filtered water, and carry your water in glass or stainless steel (water-based resin-lined) bottles rather than plastic.

- For packing lunches and snacks, use parchment, butcher paper, or wrap food in an unbleached paper towel and place in a food container.

- For water and juice storage, use glass pitchers.

- For dry food storage, use glass or stainless steel containers.

- For microwaving, use ceramic/pottery serving dishes, and cover with a plate. Serve and use a plate to cover before refrigerator storage.

- Purchase foods in glass jars to later use for storage.

Choosing safer plastic products starts with understanding the codes, found in a triangle on the bottom of the plastic containers, used to identify types of plastic:

1. **PETE (also known as PET) polyethelene terephthalate.** Used for most transparent bottles. Generally safe for use (not reuse). Generally recycled.

2. **HPDE: high-density polyethelene.** Rigid, reusable storage containers and toys. Less toxic than other plastics and recycled.

3. **PVC: polyvinyl chloride.** Plastic wraps and bottles, blister wraps. Additives in PVC are associated with birth defects and hormone-related cancers. Considered unsafe and not recycled.

4. **LDPE- low-density polyethelene.** Flexible plastic used for storage bags or wraps. Most #4 bags are not designed for reuse. Generally safe, not recycled.

5. **PPE (PP): polypropylene.** Semi-rigid plastic in squeeze bottles and yogurt tubs. Considered the safest and generally recycled.

6. **PS: polystyrene.** Throw-away utensils, rigid containers, and foam meat trays. Styrene leaches when heated. Considered toxic, not recyclable.

7. **PC: polycarbonate.** Bottles and jugs. Leaches bisphenol A, generally not safe when heated. Not generally recyclable.

Be looking for newer plant-based, biodegradable, non-petroleum plastics. Hopefully, they are coming soon!

Lurking in Your Home

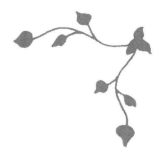

Mercury

Mercury has been shown have a negative effect on brain function and possibly suppress the immune system. Some sources of mercury you might not expect are:

> Fluorescent light bulbs,
> Batteries,

> Preservatives for vaccines and other medicines,

> Medical devices, and
> Its use in coal burning.

🌿 Please use rechargeable batteries, and recycle batteries in approved recycle sites only!

Antibacterial Soaps

Antibacterial soaps are contributing to the proliferation of antibiotic-resistant *superbugs*, which are more dangerous and also less susceptible to antibiotics when we really need them.

Teach your family good hand washing with soap. Avoid antibacterial products, or use a basic hand sanitizer containing essential oils in water!

🌿 A simple and effective hand sanitizer is adding 30 drops of lavender essential oil to 1 oz of distilled water. Store in a small flip top bottle for easy use.

🍃 In September 2016, the FDA banned 19 chemicals used in antibacterial soaps and hand sanitizers. For the complete list go to http://www.fda.gov/NewsEvents/Newsroom/PressAnnouncements/ucm517478.htm

Dry Cleaning Chemicals

PERC-chemicals used in dry cleaning are toxic to humans and animals.

🍃 Purchase washable clothing. Choose fabrics such as organic cotton or hemp, made with eco-friendly, sustainable materials.

🍃 Some clothing marked "dry clean only" may be hand washable in cold water and air dried.

Non-Stick Coatings

Teflon and other non-stick coatings on cooking and bake ware. The research remains conflicting, but a good cast iron skillet can't be beat!

🍃 Use cookware and bakeware made of stainless steel, glass, or ceramic.

🍃 If pots and pans lined with Teflon or other non-stick surface are cracked, scratched, or pitted, discontinue use!

🍃 Be cautious with antique or vintage dishes, as the glaze may be lead-based.

Flame Retardants

PDBEs are flame-retardant chemicals often used in children's sleepwear, bedding, and furniture.

🍃 Choose furniture made with organic materials whenever possible.

Phosphates

Phosphate-containing laundry products cause an overgrowth of algae in rivers and lakes, which can have serious consequences for marine life.

🍃 Make your own laundry soap with borax and baking soda, or purchase phosphate-free laundry detergents. The fish will thank you for it.

An Eco-Friendly House Is a Healthy House

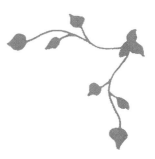

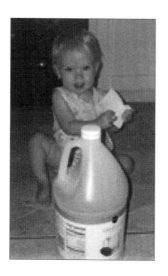

Begin with considering a more *sustainable* life style.

But what does that really mean?

It means using resources that are able to be reproduced in an environmentally healthy manner, which is respectful of the earth, as well as the plants, animals, and humans that inhabit it!

A Relatively Painless Plan

Install a water purifier and drink tap water instead of bottled water.

If all Americans used a glass or stainless steel bottle or cup for water, we could make an enormous impact on reducing the petrochemical waste.

Energy Conservation

Turn off lights when not in use, and switch to compact fluorescent light bulbs, or even better, LED (light-emitting diode) bulbs.

- If you can't buy new windows, seal off your windows and small cracks or gaps around the doors and electrical outlets.

- Reduce the temperature on your water heater by 1 to 2 degrees.

- Adjust your thermostat. Turn down the thermostat in winter, and turn up the thermostat in summer by 1 to 2 degrees. Small changes can make a big difference.

Water Conservation

- Reduce your shower time, and install a low-flow shower head and low-flow toilet flushers.

- Save laundry and dishes until there are full loads. Small loads waste water and electricity, and add pollution.

- For lawn care, use a soaker rather than traditional hoses. If you must water, do so only in the early morning to reduce evaporation.

Air Quality

- Avoid the use of plug-in or table top continuous or extended time air fresheners, which often contains phthalates. When weather is temperate, open the windows.

- *Houseplants are natural air filters.*

  - Some plants that are especially good filters:

  - **Boston Ferns** remove formaldehyde and VOCs.

- **Philodendrons, Spider Plants, and Pathos** were found to be the most efficient in the removal of formaldehyde.

- **Gerbera Daisies and Chrysanthemums** were found to be effective in the removal of benzene, a known carcinogen.

- As a rule of thumb, allow one houseplant per 100 square feet of living area. The more vigorous the plant, the more air it can filter.

- Another simple air freshening tip; take a fresh lemon and cut an "X" into the top, and place in a bowl close to the bed to allow the citrus oils to naturally freshen the air.

- Avoid, and when possible replace, PVC flooring and carpets treated with formaldehyde.

- Purchase and use only natural, organic mattresses and bedding.

- Whenever possible, begin replacing furniture made with formaldehyde-containing pressboard with furniture made with solid wood, or other alternatives, like bamboo.

- For more information on purchasing safer furniture, go to www.wellbuilding.com.

- Choose curtains and drapes made from natural organic fabrics and materials.

- When painting, avoid the toxic VOCs (volatile organic compounds), which are higher in oil baser paints. Instead, opt for water-based paints that are designated and labeled "low" or "no" VOCs.

✿ Check for radon with a simple test kit. If your home shows high levels, go to epa.gov for information on safe removal.

Personal Care Products

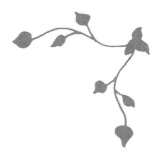

Beauty and personal care products are a huge industry in the United States. There are roughly 10,500 different chemical compounds used in these products, and sadly, only about 11% of these have been safety tested. The Environmental Working Group reports that one in every 100 personal care products contain ingredients that have been identified as human carcinogens (known to cause cancer).

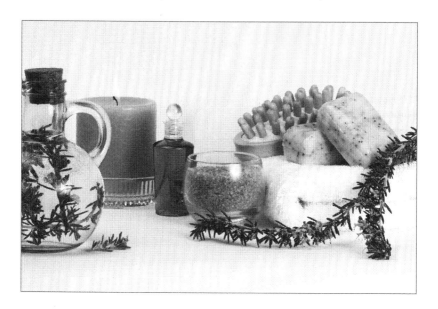

"Not so Pretty" Chemicals in Cosmetics

> **Placental extracts** in shampoos and other hair care products, which contain estrogen that is easily absorbed into the general system.

> **Pthalates,** labeled as DEHP, BBzP, or any ingredient that begins with "phth," such as phthalic acid or phthalic glycols and found in hair and skin care products, and fragrances. Pthalates have been shown to be endocrine disrupters, mimicking hormones and causing hormonal imbalances and cancer.

> **Parabens,** labeled as methyl, ethyl, proply, or butyl paraben, have been implicated in the rise of breast cancer as high levels of these compounds have been found in breast cancer tumors.

> **Aerosol propellants** in sprays contribute heavily to air pollution.

> **Aluminum by-products** in deodorants can be toxic.

> **Formalin (formaldehyde)** in nail polishes and soaps can cause serious health problems and is banned in Japan and Sweden.

> **Sodium lauryl/laureth sulfate** in shampoos, lotions, and toothpaste has been shown to damage DNA, resulting in birth defects.

> **DEA, MEA, TEA** in dyes, lotions, creams, and soaps is associated with liver and kidney cancer.

> **FD&C color pigments** are known carcinogens.

> **Fragrances** are linked to allergies and asthma, and central nervous system disorders.

> **PEG (polyethylene glycol)** removes natural oils and causes dermatitis.

> **PG (propylene glycol)** is the active ingredient in antifreeze used in deodorants. Direct contact is related to liver and kidney damage.

> **Tricolsan** is a widely used antibacterial, and is implicated in hormone disruption and immune system suppression.

> **Petrolatum** prevents the skin from breathing, and is a known carcinogen.

> **Lead** is often used in extended-wear lipsticks.

> **Toluene** in nail polishes can negatively affect the central nervous system.

Exposure to these chemicals are of particular concern with girls in puberty, as the breast tissue is developing. There is also new research into the concerns about the effects of hormone-mimicking chemicals on males. Recent research is finding lower sperm counts in men, and a general decrease in the size of newborn male genitalia.

The good news is that "green" personal care is simple and less expensive, and here is how:

🍃 Avoid synthetic dyes and coloring agents. Opting to use natural henna and herbal color agents make a much safer choice!

🍃 Many fragrances hide harmful chemicals that are not listed on the labels. To ensure the healthiest way to buy perfumes and fragrances, look for those that list the source of the scent or choose pure essential oils.

🍃 Be particularly vigilant in using these products during pregnancy and breastfeeding, and avoid or minimize the use of these products during childhood and puberty.

🍃 Purchase products with natural ingredients, avoiding phthalates and parabens whenever possible.

- Aerosol propellants: choose non-aerosol forms or those in mechanical pump bottles.

- Choose crystal or other natural deodorants, available at most health food stores.

- Rather than chemical-laden lotions, use coconut, olive, or other plant-based oils as moisturizers for face and body.

- Use natural soaps, such as castile, glycerin, or yucca plant root for shampoo, and hand and body washes.

Trusted consumer information on cosmetic safety www.SafeCosmetics.org.

To help you make decisions before purchasing products, go to www.EWG.org/skindeep to see hazard ratings on most commercially produced products. This guide makes it easy for you to buy safer products for you and your whole family.

The "Recipes" for Natural Skin and Hair Care

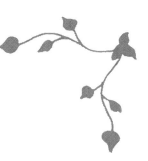

Herbal Infusions

Many recipes start with an infusion of an herb or combination of herbs. Here is the secret to creating a healing, sensuous herb infusion:

- Place 1 to 2 tablespoons dried herb, or herb combination, in 6 to 8 oz hot water.

- The herbs can be placed in the water loose, or you can use a re-usable cotton tea bag.

- Allow the herbs to "steep" for 10 to 15 minutes (if you are using roots or woody parts of the plant, steep for 20 to 23 minutes) then strain out plant material. The fragrant and medicinal qualities of the plant is infused into the water.

- This makes a great base to combine with vegetable-based soaps, butters, oils, or natural gels to make skin and hair-care products.

Basic After-Bath Splash Recipe

- 2 cups distilled water
- Heat to a steady simmer and add 2 to 3 tablespoons

dried herb or herb mixture (optional: add 1 to 2 teaspoons dried citrus fruit rind), and simmer for 20 minutes, allow to cool and strain out herbs/rinds.

- 🌿 Add 1 tablespoon each of aloe and witch hazel
- 🌿 For cooling summer splash, use lemon balm and/or lemon rinds.
- 🌿 For basic skin care splash, use lavender and chamomile.
- 🌿 For dry, inflamed skin, use calendula and yarrow.

Intensive Moisture for the Face

In 2 cups distilled hot water, steep 1 tablespoon each of dried lavender buds and chamomile flowers for 20 minutes. Strain out herbs and add:

1 oz each of lanolin and beeswax to hot water and stir until melted.

Add 3 oz avocado oil and mix well until cool.

- 🌿 Apply a small amount to clean skin and allow to soak in, 2 to 3 times weekly.

Quick, Natural After-Shower Moisturizing

- 🌿 After your shower, while your skin is still wet, apply a small amount of olive oil. Rub in well and dry as usual. Very effective for soft skin.

Basic Body Powder

1 cup corn starch

1 tablespoon each baking soda and orris root powder

🌿 Add essential oils or dried herbs, if desired.

Basic Hand and Body Lotion

¾ cup base oil (natural cold-pressed oil—olive, avocado, sweet almond, apricot kernel, jojoba, wheat germ)

1 cup aloe gel

½ cup shea, mango, or cocoa butter, softened

🌿 Mix well and add essential oils, if desired: lavender, sandalwood, chamomile, citrus, or geranium.

For a firmer hand lotion:

Warm and add ½ oz beeswax, and stir until melted and mixed well.

Basic Body Wash

1 cup liquid glycerin

½ cup floral water or herbal infusion

🌿 Mix together well, and use as a daily bath or shower cleanser.

🌿 To reduce itching, dry, or irritated skin, use a shower filter which removes chlorine and other chemicals from the shower water.

Floral Water

- Pack a clear glass jar with dried herb or herb mixture. Cover with mixture of 1 part witch hazel and 2 parts distilled water. Place in sunny window and "steep," covered and sealed for 2 weeks. Strain out herbs and store floral water in dark glass jar.

- Floral water suggestions: dried rose petals, lavender buds, chamomile flowers, or mint leaves.

Body Polish

½ cup refined sugar
2 tablespoons cold-pressed vegetable oil
5 to 7 drops of preferred essential oil

- Massage into wet skin after bath or shower and allow to soak into skin for 2 to 3 minutes before rinsing, and dry as usual.

Exfoliating Facial Scrub

1 teaspoon finely ground almonds
2 teaspoons finely ground rolled oats
1 tablespoon plain yogurt (or liquid glycerin)
1 teaspoon honey

- Mix well and apply to clean, wet skin.

- Massage in well and rinse. For best results, repeat weekly.

Dry Skin Toner

2 oz aloe gel

2 oz rose floral water

1 teaspoon each of white vinegar and witch hazel

🌿 Add contents of 1 vitamin E capsule. Apply a small amount to clean, dry skin, 2 to 3 times weekly.

Dry Skin Cleanser

2 oz aloe gel

1 teaspoon grapefruit seed extract

1 oz liquid glycerin

Optional: 10 drops lavender essential oil.

🌿 Mix well, wash and rinse, as usual.

Green Tea Toner

Heat ½ cup distilled water and steep 1 to 2 tea bags of green tea for 10 to 15 minutes.

🌿 Remove tea bags, apply to wet skin, and pat dry.

🌿 Repeat 3 to 4 times weekly.

Blemish Banish

¼ cup distilled water

½ tsp each Epsom salts and witch hazel

1 teaspoon tea-tree essential oil

🌿 Mix well and store in dark glass bottle.

🌿 Apply to clean skin as needed, 2 to 3 times daily.

Natural Herbal Shampoo

2 cups liquid castile or glycerin soap
½ cup distilled water
½ cup floral water

- Mix well and wash hair as usual.

- For dandruff control, add 5 to 7 drops of tea-tree essential oil to your daily shampoo.

Dry Scalp Conditioner

1 cup plain yogurt
10 drops rosemary essential oil

- Apply to clean hair and massage well into scalp. Allow to sit for 15 to 20 minutes and rinse thoroughly. Repeat 1 to 2 times weekly, as needed.

Conditioning After-Shampoo Rinse

2 cups floral water or herbal infusion with distilled water
1 cup white vinegar

- Apply to clean, wet hair after shampooing. Rinse and dry as usual.

Favorite hair-rinse floral waters:

> For blondes, use chamomile.

> For brunettes, use rosemary.

Natural Hand Sanitizer

1 oz distilled water

½ oz each liquid glycerin and witch hazel

Add 10 drops each of the germ-killing essential oils: lavender, tea-tree, and lemon.

🌿 Mix well and use in place of antibiotic-containing hand washes.

Nature's Face Mask

🌿 Mix together 2 oz green clay and 3 teaspoons corn flour, and store in air-tight container.

Mask Recipe

1 tablespoon clay/flour mixture

1 teaspoon finely ground rolled oats

1 teaspoon jojoba or olive oil

1 tablespoon water

3 drops lavender or chamomile essential oil

🌿 Apply a thin layer, allow to dry completely. Rinse well. Repeat weekly for best results.

Herbal Lip Balm

5 tablespoons olive oil, heat and add 1 tablespoon beeswax.

🌿 Stir until completely melted. Add 2 teaspoons of honey, and stir in 5 to 6 drops of preferred essential oil. Allow to cool and store in dark glass jar or bottle.

Natural Skin Care for Baby

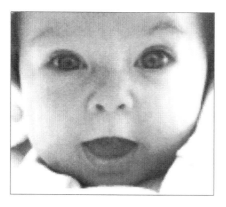

Baby Lotion

3 tablespoons olive oil
2 tablespoons coconut oil
1 teaspoon beeswax
1/4 cup distilled water
1-1/2 teaspoons glycerin

- Melt the oil and beeswax in a double boiler over medium heat. Remove from heat. Blend with an electric hand mixer until creamy.

Gentle Baby Soap

Melt 2 to 3 oz glycerin soap base.
Add 1 teaspoon aloe gel.
When slightly cooled, add 3 drops lavender essential oil.

- Place in soap mold until completely cooled.

Newborn Cord Care

🌿 Sprinkle goldenseal powder, or drops of calendula tincture, on the umbilical stump 1 to 2 times daily.

For Diaper Rash

Prepare an infusion of calendula petals (steep 1 tablespoon petals in 1 cup hot water for 10 to 15 minutes).

🌿 Allow to cool and "rinse" baby's bottom after cleaning, 3 to 4 times daily.

Or

🌿 For "yeasty" diaper rashes, add 1 teaspoon of myrrh tincture to the calendula infusion.

Baby Powder

Mix organic corn starch or arrowroot powder (about 1 cup) with 1 tablespoon each ground lavender buds or calendula petals.

🌿 Store in shaker bottle and sprinkle a small amount as needed.

Fussy-Baby Spray

1 cup distilled water
8 drops lavender essential oil

🌿 Place in spray bottle and spray on sheets, blankets, or carrier covers as needed to help soothe fussiness.

For Skin Rashes

- Apply organic aloe gel liberally to the affected area, 2 to 3 times daily or apply coconut oil liberally to affected area.

- You may want to add 3 to 5 drops of lavender or chamomile essential oil to the aloe or coconut oil.

- If you are breastfeeding, apply your milk to the diaper rash 2 to 3 times a day.

Homemade Baby Wipes

Soft cloths or wash cloths
1/4 cup natural baby shampoo
1 tablespoon olive oil
2 to 3 drops of lavender or tea-tree oil
2 cups lukewarm distilled water

- In container, mix liquid ingredients. Place on lid and tip upside down. To use, pull out from center.

Skin Rash Wash

In 2 cups hot water, add 2 teaspoons each of lavender buds, calendula petals, and linden blossoms.

- Steep for 30 minutes and strain out herbs. Cool and sponge onto affected area, 2 to 3 times daily.

- Store in dark glass jar in refrigerator.

Antiseptic Ointment

Warm 1 cup olive or infused calendula oil, and add 1/2 oz beeswax and 5 drops of vitamin E oil.

🌿 Stir well, remove from heat, and before setting up, add 15 drops lavender essential oil, 5 drops each of tea-tree and bergamot essential oils.

🌿 Store in dark bottle or jar, and use on rashes, cuts, and wounds.

Congestion Chest Rub

Warm 1 cup olive oil and add 1 to 1 1/2 oz beeswax.

🌿 Remove from heat and add 15 drops eucalyptus essential oil.

🌿 Allow to cool and set up.

🌿 Rub into chest and throat for coughs and congestion.

Sore Throat Spray

In 1 cup water, steep 2 teaspoons each horehound, mullein, and mint leaves.

🌿 Simmer for 10 to 15 minutes.

🌿 Strain and chill. Place in a spray bottle, and spray into sore throat area as needed.

Indigestion Tummy Rub

2 oz base oil

5 drops each of chamomile and fennel essential oils

🌿 Mix and massage into upper abdomen, as needed.

Soothing Infused Oil for Itch Relief

To make the infused oil:

🌿 Place dried chickweed and chamomile in a clear glass jar and pack tightly.

🌿 Cover herbs completely with a base oil: olive, sweet almond, wheat germ, apricot kernel or jojoba, and seal jar (Avoid using petroleum-based products on infants).

🌿 Place in a sunny window for 2 weeks. (Cheater's method: Place dried herbs in a slow cooker or crock pot. Cover herbs completely with base oil and cover. Simmer on low for 6 to 7 hours, and strain out herbs for a quicker infused oil.) Strain out plant material, and store infused oil in a dark glass bottle or jar.

🌿 Apply to affected area, 2 to 3 times daily.

Oatmeal Bath

🌿 Place rolled oats/oatmeal in a cotton or muslin tea bag.

🌿 Draw a comfortably warm bath and place oatmeal bag in the water for 5 minutes before placing the child in the tub to soak for 10 to 15 minutes.

Milk Bath

Milk is a soothing, moisturizing, additive that gently soothes and cleanses your child's skin. If your child is allergic to cow's milk, powdered goat's milk makes a wonderful substitute in this recipe.

 1 cup dried milk
 1/2 cup cornstarch
 2 to 3 drops lavender or chamomile essential oils (optional)

 🌿 Combine all ingredients and stir.

 🌿 To use, sprinkle 1 to 2 tablespoons in a warm bath.

Skin Cleanser (For Bath Time)

 ¼ cup Jojoba oil
 ½ cup almond oil
 10 ml honey (careful not to let babies under 12 months ingest the honey)
 2 to 3 teaspoons of oat flour

Baby Washbags Recipe

Use these wash bags as a gentle soap-free cleanser for baby.

 Place in muslin (reusable fabric tea) bags
 Lavender bud powder
 Chamomile powder
 Colloidal oatmeal fine
 Cornstarch
 A few drops of jojoba or other oil

- 🌿 Combine all the ingredients in a blender and thoroughly mix. Pour a small amount into the muslin bag.
- 🌿 When bathing baby, place bag in bath water, then gently squeeze muslin bag over baby, and rub lightly with bag.

Cradle Cap Relief

1 tablespoon olive or other cold-pressed vegetable oil
5 drops lavender pure essential oil
1 tsp aloe gel

- 🌿 Apply to affect area, and brush with a soft-bristled brush daily.

Gentle Baby Wash

2 to 3 oz organic glycerin
1 teaspoon organic aloe
1 oz herbal infusion of organic lavender or chamomile

Baby Calm Massage Oil

4 oz base oil (olive, sweet almond, jojoba, wheat germ, apricot kernel)
30 drops lavender pure essential oil
20 drops chamomile pure essential oil

- 🌿 Mix well and store in dark glass bottle.
- 🌿 Use as a gentle massage over back, belly, legs, chest, and arms.

🍂 Find out what calms more: The gentle aromatherapy or our reassuring touch. Maybe a combination of both.

Cloth Diapers: Why?

Environmental Benefits

> Disposables take 250 to 500 years to decompose.

> They are 3rd largest consumer item in landfills.

> The production of disposables each year for one baby uses over 300 lbs of wood, 50 lbs of crude oil, and 20 lbs of chlorine.

> Disposables create 60x more solid waste, and use 20x more raw materials.

Benefits to Baby

Cloth decreases exposure to harmful chemicals found in disposables such as:

> **Dioxin:** According to the EPA, dioxin is the most toxic cancer-linked chemicals.

> **Tributyltin:** Toxic chemical that can cause hormonal problems.

> **Sodium Polyacrylate:** Absorptive gel material, a similar product previously used in tampons caused toxic-shock syndrome (TSS).

Cloth is breathable, decreasing the risk of raising scrotal temperatures for boys.

Cloth costs less money than disposables.

Lawn and Garden Care

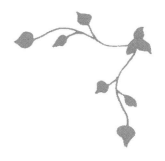

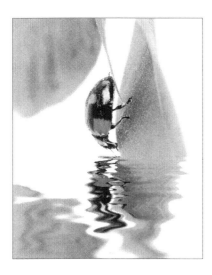

Pesticides and herbicides were among the first chemicals to be recognized as harmful to human health, and destructive to the environment. The book, *Silent Spring*, by Rachel Carson was written in the mid-1960s, and was an early warning to the dangers of these chemical compounds.

According to the EPA's own estimates, 95% of the pesticides used on residential lawns are possible, or probable, carcinogens.

Some other concerns associated with the use of herbicides and pesticides are:

> Abnormal brain activity, including hyperactivity and behavior problems in children

> Compromised brain development and learning disabilities

> Mutations to normal cells, which may result in birth defects

> Respiratory disorders and asthma in children and adults

> Toxic pollution of rivers, streams, and other waterways

> Interruption of the serotonin system, a natural way of mood balancing

How can we protect ourselves and our families from these dangers?

Call your lawn care companies and insist on the use of non-toxic, organic lawn care products. Keep your home pest-free by caulking holes, using window screens in good repair, and by using food-storage containers that easily keep out ants and other kitchen pests.

Use chemical-free substitutes for pest control, such as sprinkling garlic powder, or using cinnamon spray, in areas where ants appear.

Natural Lawn Care

🍃 For healthy, chemical-free lawns, first plant the grass that is best for your climate. In drought-prone areas, consider planting native plants and bushes instead of grass.

🍃 Don't over-mow! Keeping your grass too short promotes the growth of weeds. Keeping the grass length at least 2 to 3 inches creates a healthier lawn, naturally.

🍃 When you mow, please let the clippings fall back into the lawn, rather than clogging up landfills.

🍃 If you must water the lawn, water in the early morning only. Also, watering less often, for longer periods of time will encourage a healthier root system.

🌿 There are many ways to nourish and maintain a healthy lawn. Check with your local nurseries for organic or natural options for other lawn care products.

Gardening Nature's Way

🌿 For low-maintenance gardens, use native plants whenever possible, and plant ground cover, or use composted mulch, to stop the spread of weeds.

🌿 Herbal pest repellants, such as neem oil, garlic powder, or cayenne (hot pepper) sprays can be added to natural soaps, and sprayed on plants for effective insect control.

🌿 For more information on natural gardening, go to www.planetnatural.com for a beautiful lawn and garden you can feel good about enjoying.

🌿 Use companion planting. This means using the natural substances in the plant's roots, blooms, or flowers to repel pests and attract beneficial insects, allowing nature to do its job, creating a healthy, natural ecosystem in your yard.

Here are some beneficial plants to consider:

> **Anise** repels aphids

> **Basil** encourages better growth and flavor of tomatoes, and repels flies and mosquitoes.

> **Bay leaf,** crushed, dried, and sprinkled around your garden is a great general insecticide.

> **Catnip** deters flea beetles, aphids, squash bugs, ants, and weevils. Also deters mice and ants from the garden or in the house.

> **Chrysanthemums** kills root nematodes, and is a good general pesticide.

> **Comfrey** is a good trap crop for slugs.

> **Elderberry** is a spray made from the leaves is used against aphids, carrot root fly, cuke beetles, and peach tree borers. Leaves and small branches placed in mole runs will put them on the run.

> **Garlic** repels aphids, codling moths, Japanese beetles, root maggots, snails, and carrot root flies. It also accumulates sulfur, a natural fungicide. Concentrated garlic oils have also been shown to discourage deer from eating garden plants.

> **Lamium** repels potato bugs.

> **Lavender** repels fleas and moths. Dried sprigs, placed in closets or drawers, will discourage moths from damaging clothing.

> **Lemon balm** contains citronella compounds, a natural insect repellant.

> **Marigolds** (calendula) repels nematodes and white flies. It is often used as a weed killer as well.

> **Nasturtium** deters wooly aphids, white flies, squash bugs, cucumber beetles, and aphids.

> **Peppermint** repels white cabbage moths, aphids, and flea beetles, and is a natural insect repellant. Attracts beneficial bees.

> **Sage** repels cabbage moths, beetles, black flea beetles, and carrot flies. Sage flowers attract beneficial insects.

All Natural Fertilizers

Save and use your own compost:

> Coffee grounds for nitrogen

> Bone meal for phosphorous

> Wood ash for potassium

> Fish emulsions for nitrogen

> Cotton seed meal for nitrogen, phosphorous and potassium

> Kelp meal for potassium and abundant trace minerals

🖉 Dissolve 1 to 2 tablespoons Epsom salts in 1 gallon water, and use regularly to water plants.

🖉 Diluted beer can add the right bacteria to the soil. Combine with non-antibacterial soap to absorb well into the soil.

🖉 Compost is a great natural fertilizer. Start your compost pile now with any weeds, dead flowers, and plant-based foods (not meat or dairy).

Natural Weed Killers

🖉 Place several layers of newspapers 2 to 3 inches deep and cover with soil. Place the newspapers anywhere you want to stop the growth of weeds.

🖉 Vinegar applied directly to weeds kills them fast, but be careful where you pour. It will also kill desired vegetation.

- Another effective weed killer is salt, poured directly on the unwanted weed. Same caution applies!
- Boiling water is another way to rid driveways, sidewalks, and patios of unwanted bloomers.
- Many natural weed-killing products contain vinegar, salt, clove, or citrus oil.

An inexpensive, effective natural weed killer is:

1 oz each of vodka, liquid detergent, and vinegar.

- Mix well and spray on unwanted plants or vegetation. Reapply as needed.

You can be the best weed killer. Pulling weeds is great exercise.

Natural Pesticide Plants

> Pyrethium	> Sage	> Peppermint
> Marigold	> Nasturtium	> Basil
> Catnip	> Lemon Balm	> Garlic

Beneficial Bug Attractants (ladybugs)

> Cilantro	> Fennel	> Sage
> Dill	> Yarrow	> Dandelion

Herbal Infusions for Bug Zapping

- Heat 1 quart of water to simmering.
- Add ¼ cup each dried garlic, rhubarb, and cayenne pepper.

- Simmer for 15 to 20 minutes and remove herbs.
- Place in spray bottles and spray daily as needed to keep pests away.

For more information, go to www.treehugger.com

Keeping Biting/Stinging Bugs Away

- Mosquitoes are most active at dusk and dawn. Limit outside activities at these times.
- Wear long sleeves and long pants whenever possible.
- Camouflage yourself. Wear clothes that blend with your surroundings.
- Avoid the use of perfumes or colognes, hair spray, or scented deodorants.
- Remove any standing water in pools, bird baths, gutters, or rain water-collection containers.
- Some evidence states that eating bananas, peanuts, or chocolate can attract mosquitoes.
- Soy bean oil has natural insect repellant properties.
- Place vanilla beans around tables and chairs to ward off bugs.

Natural Insect Repellant

4 oz water (with a splash or witch hazel) or 4 oz soy bean oil
Add 20 drops citronella essential oil and
15 drops each lavender, eucalyptus, and lemon

🌿 Mix well and place in spray bottle. Apply to skin while outdoors, as needed. Safe for children over 12 months of age.

Other Helpful Essential Oils

Note: Always dilute essential oils before applying to the skin. The general rule is this:

1 oz base oil or water and add no more than 20 to 30 drops of essential oil or combination of oils.

🌿 For pregnant women, young children, or persons in poor health, reduce the amount to no more than 20 drops of essential oil per ounce on base oil or water (see dilution chart in aromatherapy section).

🌿 To ward off ticks, use rose geranium, bay, eucalyptus, or lavender.

🌿 For pesky mosquitoes, use lemon, citronella, thyme or lavender.

🌿 To repel flies, use lavender, eucalyptus, peppermint, or cedar.

🌿 To keep fleas away, use orange or citronella.

Feeding
Our Families

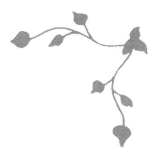

Hippocrates, the father of medicine, gave us real wisdom in 400 BC: *Let food be your medicine – let medicine be your food.*

We, in this modern society, must be a real disappointment to him. Not only is food no longer our first line of medicine, it is responsible for causing "unhealth."

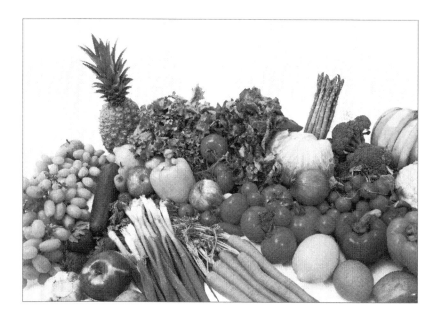

Breastfeeding

Breastfeeding is the best first food! Encourage and support breastfeeding to promote health and prevent disease.

Some good reasons to breastfeed:

For Mothers

> Less incidence of breast and ovarian cancer

> Lower rates of osteoporosis

> Reduced risk of cardiovascular disease

For Babies

> Reduced risk of allergies and asthma

> Reduced risk of obesity and diabetes

> Reduced risk of SIDS, childhood leukemia, diarrhea, and upper respiratory and other infections.

Other benefits include less worktime missed for parents, less environmental waste, and higher IQ scores.

With all those benefits, what can we do to help new mothers get started in breastfeeding?

1. Encourage early and uninterrupted skin-to-skin contact between mother and newborn in the first hours and days after birth.

2. Have mothers talk with their care providers to assure the first feeding within the first 1 to 2 hours after birth.

3. Avoid supplementation with formula unless medically necessary. Exclusive breastfeeding is the best choice, whenever possible.

4. Educate mothers and new families about normal newborn feeding and sleeping patterns.

5. Give mothers names and numbers of support resources in the community for breastfeeding support.

Food Supply

All too often, naturally occurring foods are refined, processed, colored, preserved, emulsified, modified, packaged, and marketed. It is actually hard to find real food, sometimes.

As our foods became more processed, and able to stay stable for longer periods of time to accommodate transportation and extended shelf storage in stores, the need to add artificial ingredients increased, and food became more of a commodity than nourishment.

The proliferation of *quick and easy, convenient,* and *able to eat on the run* foods was appealing, and at first, we followed the program, not questioning the consequences of altering our basic foods. But at what cost to our health is this convenience?

Fortunately, the winds of change are in the air. Consumer-driven change is often the best and most enduring, and that's the trend we are seeing now.

Some Common Food Additives of Concern

> Aspartame/artificial sweeteners
> Sodium benzoate
> Nitrates/nitrites
> MSG
> Artificial and some "natural" flavors
> Potassium bromate
> Hormones
> Colors and dyes
> Sulphur dioxide
> BHA/BHT
> Genetically modified foods

Some of the More troubling food additives

> **Trans-fats (hydrogenated/partially hydrogenated oils),** and newer interestified fats (stearatic acids),

which are added to foods to increase shelf life, but have been shown to cause inflammation, are associated with heart disease, and may be implicated in cancer.

> **High fructose corn syrup.** This really satisfies the insatiable American sweet tooth. Unfortunately, it is also adding to the obesity concerns, as well as rising rates of diabetes.

> **Artificial dyes and colorings** have been added to many processed foods to make them more visually appealing, often more appealing to children. Many studies since the 1970s have linked behavior problems and learning inabilities to the artificial dyes and colors in foods. Children given a preservative/dye-free diet have been shown to demonstrate a significant improvement in behavior and learning.

> **Genetically modified foods.** Oh, my! Splicing the DNA of a carp and a tomato should make everyone's blood run cold, but many look to this science with hope and admiration. Biotechnology foods are in the marketplace now. Unfortunately, this science has been unleashed on the public without sufficient research done to assure its safety. Looks a little like the American public is the experiment. Many are asking for the right to know which of our family's foods are being genetically modified. Let us make an informed choice!

> **Hormones in the meat and dairy.** Many growth and estrogen-like hormones are added to animal feed, which makes them a little "fluffier" for a "fluffier" price at market. Unfortunately, these estrogen-like and growth hormones are implicated in the rising

rates of reproductive cancers in males and females, along with other reproductive concerns, such as early puberty, menstrual and menopausal dysfunctions, and infertility concerns.

> **Chemical preservatives.** Labeled in many ways, names, letters, and numbers. The best advice is if you can't pronounce it, don't eat it!

> **Bleached and enriched.** This "process" is the most confusing of all. Strip the naturally occurring foods of their nutrients, then replace them with artificial vitamins? Go figure!

> **Herbicide and pesticide residues.** Once you make the switch to clean, chemical-free foods, you'll notice the improvement in the taste, aroma, and color, and the reduced worry over the effects of the chemicals can be so freeing!

Want more info? Go to www.organic-center.org

Many of these, and other additives, are implicated in behavior problems, asthma, reproductive disorders, or cancers. For more information and food health ratings go to http://www.ewg.org/foodscores/

What Do We Do Now?

We need to rethink our relationship with food, which has become a necessary evil, an inconvenience, and a drudge.

Food is nourishment for our bodies and souls. Food preparation can be a memory, a social event, and a gift. Sitting together at the family table to share a meal is now a rare occurrence, rather than an integral part of family communication.

The most basic building blocks of health have been turned into marketing tricks and clever jingles.

On your next trip to the food market or grocery, take a few extra minutes to really look at what is available:

> Organic produce?
> Hormone-free meats and dairy?
> Healthier snack options, like hummus?

> Pastas and breads made with whole, unrefined grains?
> Healthy sources of fats?

It can be a challenge and a reward to rediscover the kitchen again. Build some traditions and memories with family recipe foods, and make the family table a priority, at least for a few times a week.

Choose organic foods whenever possible. The more we purchase these products, the more we support not only our own health, but the health of the planet as well.

Skip the artificial sweeteners, and opt for honey, stevia, agave, black strap molasses, date sugar, and coconut sugar.

According to The Environmental Working Group, the foods most heavily contaminated with herbicides and pesticides are as follows. Spending a bit more money on organic versions of these *dirty dozen* foods is worth the extra expense.

> Strawberries
> Apples
> Nectarines
> Peaches
> Celery
> Grapes

> Cherries
> Spinach
> Tomatoes
> Sweet bell peppers
> Cherry tomatoes
> Cucumbers

The "Clean 15" foods tend to be less contaminated:

> Avocados

> Sweet Corn

> Pineapples

> Cabbage

> Sweet peas (frozen)

> Onions

> Asparagus

> Mangos

> Papayas

> Kiwi

> Eggplant

> Honeydew Melon

> Grapefruit

> Cantaloupe

> Cauliflower

Read labels! When you see long lists of ingredients that are difficult to pronounce, they are also probably hard to digest.

Healthy, Family-Friendly Foods

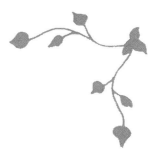

Smoothies

Blend your favorite fresh or frozen fruits and veggies in organic cow's milk, or milk substitutes, such as soy, rice, hemp, or almond milks.

- 🌿 For extra nutrition, add flax seed meal, chia seeds, brewer's yeast, or 1 to 2 teaspoons of spirulina or chlorophyll.

Make-Your-Own Granola

4 cups rolled oats

1 cup wheat germ

1/4 cup each, raw or toasted, nuts and seeds

1/2 cup raisins or fried fruit

1/2 cup warmed honey

- 🌿 Mix dry ingredients well and add honey stir until moistened.

- 🌿 Place on baking sheet and allow to cool.

Kids Love Peanut Butter

Read labels; many commercial peanut butters contain trans-fats.

- Choose natural peanut butters, or opt for almond butter instead.

Choosing Dairy

- For hormone balancing at any age, use only organic milk, and look for cheeses and yogurts made only with organic milk.

Breads and Cereals

- The choice is simple—use only whole-grain breads.
- Read the label, not the advertising on the front.
- Look for whole wheat, rye, oat, bulgur, barley, or quinoa.

Seedy Subjects

Seeds are a great source of vitamins and fiber

Easy Sesame Spread

3/4 cup natural toasted sesame seeds
1 tablespoon honey
¼ to 1/2 cup organic apple juice
Pinch of salt

🌿 Grind seeds in blender or coffee grinder. Add other ingredients and stir until consistency is thick. Use as a dip for veggies or as spread for whole-grain crackers.

The Sweet Tooth

To sweeten foods or drinks, use:

> Sugar in the raw   > Molasses
> Stevia   > Brown rice syrup
> Agave
> Honey (not for babies
>   under 12 months of age)

Look for foods that contain these natural sweeteners, rather than using refined sugar or artificial sugar substitutes.

Quick, Easy Snacks

Try hummus. It comes in garlic, dill, sundried tomato and many more. Scoop the hummus with whole-grain chips, like blue corn, for a healthy, fast snack anytime.

Roasted Seeds

Raw pumpkin, sesame, or any kind of seed can be oven-roasted with your favorite natural seasonings.

🌿 Place a thin layer of your seeds on a baking sheet. Sprinkle with seasonings and bake at 200 degrees for about 10 to 15 minutes, or until golden brown. Store in an airtight container.

For Heart Health

Avoid all trans-fats, and limit saturated animal fats. Switch to a more plant-based diet with more fruits, vegetables, and healthy fats, such as avocado and coconut oils.

- Plan on cooking with olive oil as much as possible, and use garlic as much as possible in foods.

Blood Sugar Balancing

Eat low on the food chain.

Increase fiber foods: oatmeal, whole-grain cereals and breads, seeds, and vegetables.

Cook with spices known to balance blood sugar:

> Cinnamon > Cloves

> Bay leaf > Turmeric

Herbs used for blood sugar control:

> Fenugreek > Gymnema > Spirulina

> Bitter melon > Prickly pear

Mood-Balancing Foods

- Add omega 3s: flax, hemp seed, salmon, walnuts.
- Include foods rich in B vitamins: watercress, kale, peas, bananas.
- Include foods rich in magnesium: cashews, kelp, wheat bran.
- Water, water, water!

Foods to Reduce Inflammation

Include these foods in your daily nutrition plan.

- Omega 3 foods: flax seeds/meal, walnuts, and salmon
- Dark cherries, pineapple, mango, and blueberries
- Dark green leafy vegetables
- Medicinal mushrooms, including maitake and reishi
- Tea: especially green or white
- Fermented vegetables and foods
- Garlic for cooking and as a condiment
- Legumes: lentils, chickpeas

Spices to Reduce Inflammation

Use these regularly to season foods or as teas, tinctures, or capsules.

| > Ginger | > Rosemary | > Oregano |
| > Turmeric | > Cloves | |

Foods to Avoid or Minimize

- Highly processed prepackaged meals and foods
- Refined carbohydrates in breads and pastas
- Cured/processed meats and full-fat dairy
- Margarines and spreads containing trans/hydrogenated fats
- Refined white sugar and white flour
- Regular, large consumption of alcohol

For Good General Health

- Make your foods colorful!
- Lots of green, yellow, red, purple, and blue are found in a variety of fruits and vegetables every day.

Eat low on the food chain

- The majority of your daily foods should be fruits, veggies, nuts, seeds, and whole grains.
- Think of meat and dairy as a condiment-size portion only, not the main attraction.
- Choose whole foods in their natural state whenever possible.

Power Foods

Foods to include in your diet regularly:

- Almonds
- Flax and chia seeds
- Garlic
- Mushrooms
- Ginger
- Wild caught salmon
- Kiwi
- Tomatoes
- Carrots
- Sea vegetables
- Apples
- Coconut
- Green Tea
- Broccoli
- Olive oil
- Pomegranate
- Mango
- Bananas
- Whole soy: tofu, miso
- Walnuts
- Kefir
- Avocado

> Algae: green, brown, or
> blue-green
> Colorful berries:

raspberries, blueberries,
strawberries

Read labels. Take action. Talk to your local grocer and request healthier, organic foods to be made available.

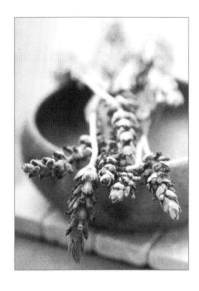

Natural Basic Family Care

Please consult your health care provider before beginning any new therapies.

For improved general good health, make a commitment to spend time outdoors with your family.

Being in nature has been shown to:

> Reduce levels of stress hormones, lessen depression.
> Improve quality of sleep.
> Encourage release of serotonin, our "happy hormone" for better moods.
> Make exercise easier and more enjoyable.
> Lower symptoms of ADHD in children.
> Improve mental clarity and focus.
> Promote creativity.

> Lower health-related problems in older people.

> Boost in energy levels with as little as 20 minutes per day out of doors.

> Perform better on memory-related tests.

> Reduce signs and symptoms of inflammation.

> Enhance immune system function.

> Reduce risk of developing nearsightedness (myopia).

In addition, sun exposure is known to be the best source of vitamin D.

So plan some time outdoors: playing, gardening, hiking or walking, picnicking, washing the car, volunteering to get neighbors and family members who may have physical concerns outside regularly, relaxing or reading outside, or collecting flowers for indoor aromatherapy.

Make nature a part of your life for a healthier family.

Minor Injuries

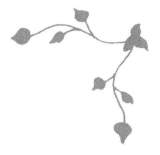

> **Honey** is the oldest "antibiotic." Apply to cuts, scratches, and other wounds to prevent infection and speed healing (Babies under 1 year of age cannot eat the honey).

> **Yarrow** is nature's bandage. Fresh or dried leaves applied directly to the wound will reduce bleeding and prevent infection.

> **Calendula** petals made into an infusion. Steep 1 tablespoon in 6 to 8 oz of hot water for 10 to 15 minutes. Apply to any wound 2 to 3 times a day to speed healing and prevent infection.

> **Black walnut tincture** can be applied directly to any wound to prevent bacterial, viral, or fungal infections.

> **Goldenseal powder** can be sprinkled on wounds to speed healing.

> **Natural aspirin:** white willow bark, meadowsweet, and vervain. These can be taken by older children and adults as teas, tinctures, or in capsule form.

Antiseptic Wash

½ cup each distilled water and apple cider vinegar
10 drops each lavender and tea-tree essential oils
1 teaspoon honey

- Blend well and apply to wounds or rashes. Store in dark glass bottle or jar.

To make a natural, healing salve

- Begin with a calendula infused oil.
- Pack dried petals in a clear glass jar and completely cover the herbs with a base oil, such as olive or sweet almond. Allow to sit in sunny window for 2 weeks and strain out herbs or use the cheater's method by placing the dried calendula petals in a slow cooker or crock pot and simmer on low for 6 to 7 hours, and then strain out herbs.
- Warm 1 ½ cups infused oil, add 1 oz beeswax, and allow to slowly melt. Once the wax is completely melted, pour warm oil mixture into dark bottle or jar to harden to a firm salve.
- Use on cuts, wounds, scratches, or rashes, 2 to 3 times daily as needed.

For Headache Relief

To 1 oz base oil, add 10 to 12 drops each of lavender and peppermint essential oils. Mix well and massage into temples or back of the neck as needed to relive headaches.

Or

Combine 10 drops each of lavender and peppermint essential oils. Place a small amount on a cotton ball and inhale vapors as needed.

For Minor Burns and Sunburns

- Apply aloe vera gel directly to the burn. Chill for cooling relief.

- Steep 1 black or green tea bag in 6 to 8 oz hot water for 10 minutes. Remove tea bag and liberally apply tea infusion to the burn area every 2 to 3 hours.

- For soothing burns, apply plain yogurt to the area for 10 to 15 minutes, 2 to 3 times a day, as needed.

- Crushed raw potato placed in a moistened cloth and applied to the burn will relieve pain and cool the burn.

- Undiluted lavender essential oil can be applied directly to the burn, 2 to 3 times daily.

For Indigestion and Heartburn

- Steep 1 teaspoon fennel seeds in 6 to 8 oz hot water for 10 minutes. Strain out the seeds and sweeten with honey. Drink 1 to 2 cups as needed.

- Include probiotics and fermented foods, like kefir, in your daily nutrition plan.

- Other herbal teas that can help are catnip, lemon balm, peppermint, marjoram, or ginger.

- Herbal bitters are herbs that increase digestive juices: gentian, dandelion, and wild lettuce.

- Foods that assist with digestion: almonds, garlic, olives, walnuts, apples, fennel seeds, and papaya.

- Spices that assist with digestion: basil, bay, allspice, caraway, chives, coriander, dill, nutmeg, parsley, and cinnamon.

- For long-term indigestion, try slippery elm capsules 1 to 2 times daily, as needed.
- For indigestion with diarrhea, drink 1 to 2 cups of red raspberry tea.

Tummy-Tamer Tea

- Combine 1 tablespoon each of ginger slices, red raspberry leaf, peppermint leaf, and ½ tsp ground cinnamon. Combine and store in dark glass jar.
- When needed, add 1 to 2 teaspoon of herb mixture, and steep in 6 to 8 oz hot water for 5 to 10 minutes. Strain out herbs and sweeten with honey.
- Drink 1 to 2 cups as needed for indigestion.
- Essential oils can be diffused in the air or placed on a cotton ball for inhalation to relieve indigestion.

Oils that Reduce Indigestion

> Basil
> Bergamot
> Chamomile
> Cinnamon
> Clove
> Fennel
> Ginger
> Lemongrass
> Rosemary
> Sage
> Thyme

For Colds and Flu

Echinacea, in tincture or capsule form, should be taken at the onset of symptoms and continued until symptoms are gone. Taking Echinacea will not prevent colds, but it has been shown to reduce the severity and length of symptoms. At onset of symptoms, eat a raw clove of **garlic** to kill the cold or flu virus.

Elderberry tea has been used for centuries to relieve the symptoms of the flu, aching, and respiratory congestion. Drink 2 to 3 cups a day until symptoms disappear.

For coughs and chest congestion, prepare a cup of mullein tea with 1 to 2 teaspoons of **dried mullein leaf or flower**. Steep 10 minutes and sweeten with a natural sweetener. Drink 3 to 4 cups a day to relieve coughing.

To clear congestion and assist in killing upper respiratory bacteria or viruses, try a **eucalyptus steam**. Place 1 to 2 inches of water in a small pan in the stove. Heat to simmering and add 6 to 8 drops of eucalyptus to the simmering water. Deeply inhale the steam until the aroma evaporates. Repeat 3 to 4 times daily, as needed.

Herbal teas that have expectorant qualities: horehound, mullein, hyssop, thyme, and wild cherry.

Herbal Chest Rub

Warm ½ cup olive oil and add ½ oz beeswax, stir on low heat, until beeswax is completely melted. Remove from heat and add 30 drops eucalyptus pure essential oil, and 10 drops each lavender and peppermint essential oils. Pour into dark glass jar to cool.

🌿 Apply gently to upper chest and throat twice daily to reduce congestion and coughing.

For Cold Sores

At the onset of the tingling of a cold sore, dab a small amount of tea-tree essential oil directly on the cold sore, and repeat 4 to 5 times a day until it disappears.

🌿 Drink 2 to 3 cups of lemon balm tea to also stop cold sores fast.

For Warts

For warts on feet or hands, place 1 to 2 drops of tea-tree oil on the wart and cover with duct tape. Keep covered for 3 to 4 days. Remove tape. Repeat as needed until wart is gone.

Three System Healing

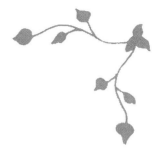

To promote good general health, keep these 3 systems in good working order and the rest of your body will thank you!

1. **Digestive Tract.** Without a healthy digestive tract, we don't absorb our nutrients.

    > Avoid additives, preservatives, and refined food as much as possible.

    > Remember, the closer to the natural form of the food, the more easily recognized and used it is by the body.

    > Acidophilus, fermented foods, and probiotics help to keep the correct bacterial balance for the best digestion of foods.

    > Include high-nutrient foods, like the supergreen foods, as much as possible (spirulina, kelp, barley grass, and alfalfa).

2. **Liver.** This powerful organ keeps our body detoxified and clean.

    > Reduce exposures to environmental contaminants.

    > Increase raw vegetables and fruits.

    > Add liver supporting herbs: milk thistle and dandelion as teas, tinctures, and capsules.

3. **Immune System**. This system provides the ability to defend against disease.

> Back to basics: nutrition, exercise, and lifestyle is the best immune-system booster.

> Include medicinal mushrooms, such as shiitake, maitake, and reishi.

> Consider teas daily with the blood-cleansing herbs: burdock or red clover.

> Or immune-stimulant herbs, especially during cold and flu season, or during times of emotional or physical distress: astragalus, rhodiola, ginseng, and cat's claw.

Reducing Stress, Naturally

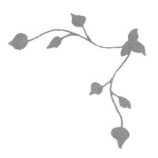

Two-Minute Relaxation

- Get comfortable. Close your eyes. Imagine a peaceful forest with cascading waterfalls and gentle warm breezes. Let your body relax.

- Breathe deeply, in through your nose, out through your mouth. As you exhale, imagine the tension leaving your body with each breath. Let the joys of your life surround you.

Stress-Busting Strategies

Calming Herbal Teas

Steep 1 to 2 teaspoon herb, or herb mixture, in 6 to 8 oz hot water for 5 to 10 minutes. Sweeten, if desired, with natural sweetener, like honey.

- Herbs that promote relaxation: chamomile, lemon balm, passionflower, valerian, skullcap, oatstraw, catnip, and hops.

- Relax and drink a cup whenever you need some calming.

Aromatherapy

Essential oils can be diffused into the air, 10 to 15 drops added to a bath, diluted in a massage oil (20 to 30 drops in 1 oz base oil), or diluted in water as a mister. Alternatively, place 3 to 5 drops on a cotton ball or aromastone to keep at your desk or bedside.

- Essential oils known to have a relaxing effect: lavender, chamomile, rose, geranium, ylang ylang, patchouli, sandalwood, and clary sage.
- Essential oils that are uplifting: citrus (lemon, orange, tangerine), bergamot, peppermint, neroli, and rosemary.

Exercise

- Exercise is a natural antidepressant. It encourages release of mood-elevating hormones. Exercise outdoors, when possible; 10 to 15 minutes of sun exposure can also encourage mood-stabilizing hormones.

Breath Work

- Use your breath for relaxation. Sit quietly and focus on each breath without changing the rate or rhythm. Become aware of how each breath feels as you take it in and out of the nose, through the lungs.
- Now begin to change your breathing pattern to slow, deliberate, quiet breaths, in through the nose and exhaled through the mouth.
- With each exhalation, allow the muscles to release tension. With each breath out, breathe the tension away.

Use Your 5 Senses to Help Relax

Use the power of the mind-body connection to imagine soothing, calming images. Allow those recalled feelings to release physical and emotional tension.

> **Taste:** Herbal teas, chocolate, family comfort foods, cold lemonade on a hot day or hot cocoa on a cold day, fresh baked bread.

> **Smell:** Aromatherapy, freshly mowed grass, air after a rain, dinner cooking, cookies baking, babies, scents that evoke your favorite memories.

> **Hearing:** Ocean waves or gentle rain, white noise, soothing music, wind through the trees, familiar voices, or laughter.

> **Touch:** Hug or caress, pet's fur, warm bath water, soft blankets and comforters, walking barefoot in the grass, velvety flowers, or a cool breeze on a hot day.

> **Sight:** The sunrise or sunset, lush green fields, colorful flowers, misty mountains, moonlight reflecting of new snow, changing fall leaves, friends and family smiles, rainbows, or your favorite color.

Aromatherapy for Natural Calming and Healing

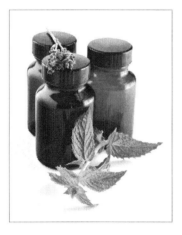

I love using the essential oils. It's a great way to incorporate "plant power" in our everyday lives. You can use the essential oils for chemical-free cleaning (and you get that uplifting feeling), gentler skin and hair care, physical healing for wounds and rashes, and emotional balancing. What great tools to keep around!

But like so many other things, you need to be aware of some precautions before using these concentrated plant oils and essences.

Using Essential Oils Safely

- Do not take internally.
- Use orally only under supervision of credentialed health care provider. *Toxicities are common with oral intake.*
- *You rarely need internal use for beneficial effects.*
- *Do not use orally with children, pregnant women, or compromised adults.*
- Use only small amount: drops.

- 🍃 Use only approved oils for children or pregnant women, in correct dilution.
- 🍃 Dilute before applying topically (except lavender and tea-tree.)

Safe Dilutions

1 oz base or infused oil. Add 20 to 30 drops essential oil or combination of oils for healthy adults.

For pregnancy	15 to 20 drops
For children	12 to 15 drops
For babies	10 to 12 drops
For health compromised	15 to 20 drops

- 🍃 Apply to affected/targeted area 2 to 3 times daily.

Common Base (Carrier) Oils to Mix with Your Essential Oils

> **Sweet almond:** Light to medium weight; moisturizing; all skin types

> **Apricot kernel:** Lightweight; healing; all skin types

> **Avocado:** Heavy weight; rich in vitamins; slight sunscreen; all skin types. Good for mature, damaged skin.

> **Coconut:** Solid at room temperature; melts on the skin; may cause allergic reaction.

> **Grapeseed:** Lightweight; may cause acne.

> **Jojoba:**   Medium weight; much like the body's sebum; good for dry skin.

> **Olive oil:**   Medium to heavy weight; nourishing; slight color and scent; healing; regenerating.

🌿 Use only pure essential oils.

🌿 Do not use in or near the eyes.

🌿 Use extra care on broken skin.

Essential Oils to Avoid

> Bitter almond
> Buchu
> Camphor
> Rue
> Clove
> Tansy

> Mugwort
> Wintergreen
> Pennyroyal
> Wormwood
> Sassafras

Here's how to use them wisely.

🌿 Add 10 to 15 drops of oil to your bath to relax before bedtime.

🌿 Place 20 to 30 drops in 1 oz base oil (olive, sweet almond, jojoba) for massaging oils and healing skin wounds and rashes.

🌿 Place 3 to 5 drops on a cotton ball and leave on desk or night stand to inhale the magic.

🌿 Add 2 to 3 drops in daily shower gel or shampoo.

🌿 Put 4 to 5 drops in a cup of warm or cool water. Dip cloth for a topical compress for topical healing like muscle or joint pains.

🌿 Add to electric, lamp ring, or candle diffusers to diffuse in the air to relax or invigorate.

🌿 Add 5 to 8 drops to a pan of simmering water for a steam to clear respiratory congestion.

Common Essential Oils and Their Uses

> **Bergamot:** Citrus-like, uplifting, antiseptic, and cleansing

> **Cedarwood:** Musky, earthy aroma, great antiseptic for the respiratory tract

> **Chamomile:** Calming, reduces tensions, soothing to irritated skin

> **Clary sage:** Earthy tone, emotionally and spiritually balancing

> **Eucalyptus:** Clears sinus and respiratory congestion

> **Geranium:** Strongly floral, antidepressant, and hormone balancing

> **Lavender:** Relaxing, enhances sleep, reduces headache pain, healing to wounds

> **Patchouli:** Musky aroma, quieting, anti-inflammatory properties

> **Peppermint:** Uplifting, invigorating, reduces stomach upset

> **Rosemary:** Supports mental clarity, focus and intuition, relieves aching muscles

> **Sandalwood:** Used in rituals of meditation, moisturizing to the skin

> **Tangerine:** Soothes and calms, cooling, reduces digestive upsets

> **Tea-tree:** Antiseptic, used for acne, and fungal skin infections

> **Ylang Ylang:** Relaxing, encourages sleep, stimulates the immune system

How to Start a More Natural, Greener Life: Begin at Home

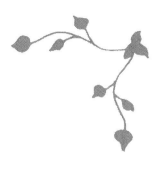

Start by taking an inventory around your home. Don't panic. It's already made for you on the next page.

This time, read labels with a newly educated eye for environmental and your family's health. Look carefully for:

> Toxic chemicals you thought were giving you a cleaner home.

> Personal care products that you now know are dangerous. Not pretty!

> Foods that are prepared with health-robbing ingredients, such as trans-fats, artificial sweeteners, GMOs, chemical dyes, and preservatives.

> Lawn and garden care products, such as polluting herbicides and pesticides that are creating a crisis in our environment, as well as serious health concerns for our children.

> Make a plan and a promise to begin purchasing energy-efficient appliances.

Step Two is replacing toxic, health-robbing products with clean, health-giving products all around the house, inside and out!

Make a shopping list including the natural ingredients you can use for simple, green cleaning: vinegar (by the gallon!), baking soda, and lemon juice.

Schedule a party with your family and friends to create your own healthy skin and hair care products. Purchase organic herbs and essential oils, some butters and oils, and start a new trend with fun, simple ways to beautiful, glowing skin, and healthy, shiny hair.

Support local, organic farmers whenever possible. Ask you grocer about making more healthful foods available.

Step Three is to talk to people, schools, churches, and civic groups. Spread the word about how important and easy it is to begin a more natural, greener life!

Cleaning Up My Little Corner of the World: a Checklist to Begin a Green Home

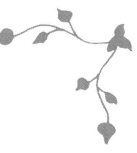

Home Chemical Inventory

ROOM	FOUND	REMOVED	REPLACED
Bathroom			
> Caustic toilet bowl cleaner	☐	☐	☐
> Chemical cleaners	☐	☐	☐
Personal Care Products			
> Parabens	☐	☐	☐
> Laureth sulfates	☐	☐	☐
> Fragrances	☐	☐	☐
> PEGs	☐	☐	☐
> Phthalates	☐	☐	☐
> Antimicrobials/triclosan	☐	☐	☐
> Others	☐	☐	☐

ROOM	FOUND	REMOVED	REPLACED
Lawn and Garden			
> Chemical herbicides	☐	☐	☐
> Chemical pesticides	☐	☐	☐
> Others	☐	☐	☐
Kitchen			
> Trans-fats	☐	☐	☐
> Artificial sweeteners	☐	☐	☐
> Hormone-containing meats and dairy	☐	☐	☐
> Food dyes or colorings	☐	☐	☐
> GMO foods	☐	☐	☐
> Non-stick PFC coated cookware	☐	☐	☐
> Plastic food prep/ storage containers	☐	☐	☐
> Others	☐	☐	☐

Be Kind to the Earth: the Whole "Green" Picture

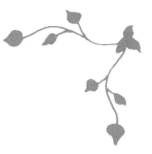

How to: Reduce ❯ Reuse ❯ Recycle ❯ Repair

For local resources for recycling and safe disposal of hazardous substances, visit www.earth911.org

> No disposable cleaning products. Please reuse towels, sheets, and washcloths for cleaning, dusting, or car washing.

> Wash or rinse aluminum foil for reuse.

> Rechargeable batteries. Re-use many times before disposal.

> Swap tools and equipment with neighbors and friends.

> Share books with friends or your neighborhood book club.

> Repair kitchen appliances, sew or darn clothing that can be repaired, or donate clothing, small appliances, dishes, toys, and other household items.

> Purchase energy-saving appliances.

> Purchase power. Choose *green* companies for purchasing or investing.

> Ban the Bag. Use canvas/reusable bags for shopping to reduce environmental plastics.

> Forego meat once a week, and choose sustainable vegetables for meals.

> Wrap presents in Sunday's comics or reusable towels, or re-use gift bags.

> Make planting trees and plants a family activity.

Reducing your Carbon Footprint

> For every degree you lower your thermostat (for heating), you cut energy by 3%; 5 degrees can save 3,150 lbs of CO_2 emissions.

> Putting your computer to sleep for 12 hours a day can save 576 lbs of CO_2 annually ($44).

> Replacing 5 light bulbs with compact fluorescents can save about 500 lbs of CO_2.

> For every 10 degrees you reduce your water heater temperature, you reduce CO_2 emissions by 3% to 5%, saving 733 lbs of CO_2.

Resources for Further Reading and Action Plans

🌿 **HealthyChild.org**

🌿 **AAEMonline.org** (American Academy of Environmental Medicine)

🌿 **Organic-Center.org**

🌿 **EWG.org** (The Environmental Working Group)

🌿 **NRDC.org** (Natural Resources Defense Council)

🌿 **toxnet.nlm.nih.gov/cgi-bin/sis/htmlgen?TRI** (Toxic Release Inventory)

🌿 **toxnet.nlm.nih.gov/cgi-bin/sis/htmlgen?CCRIS** Chemical Carcinogenesis Research Information System (CCRIS)

🌿 **sis.nlm.nih.gov/enviro/envirohealthlinks.html** (Enviro-Health Links)

🌿 **cerhr.niehs.nih.gov/** (Center for the Evaluation of Risks to Human Reproduction/NIEHS)

Made in the USA
Charleston, SC
22 February 2017